I admire Amanda Lera's honesty of her journey and her approach to resolving her challenges. This is an enlightening read with positive messages, which the reader can find relief from their stress in the moment.

   – Dan Brooks, Founder of GiveUpPain.com and author of *Fear, Phobias and Freedom* Co-founder of The Feeling Path ILLUMINATED, a transformational journey

Amanda's work, reflection and confidence are an inspiration. This books acknowledgment of difficult times and the effects on the body, are undeniably relatable in so many ways. Admiration, Inspirational, a true understanding of the need to change oneself, is to scalp oneself to be true.

   – Beverley Morris-Turbitt, Developmental Service Worker

Amanda's words inspire me in every part of life. *If I'm so Zen, Why Is My Hair Falling Out?* is motivational. I didn't realize truly how I was being affected until I read this book. It has helped me to harness my self-awareness and empowerment. I can assure you, from now on I will only pour from my overflow. Thank you for being real, honest and inspirational.

   – Christina Vecia, Owner of Lindeza Spa House

WOW. Such a beautiful book. Without a doubt made me think completely differently about my entire experience with hair loss.

Amanda has done a beautiful job in not only writing but also guiding you through this story. She provides you with so many real world examples which make it very easy to follow and understand. You can feel the love flowing from her words as you move through her book and start to turn your attention inwards. The tools that she provides you with are absolutely life changing and when you start to implement them, you will feel the difference. This is a phenomenal resource to have at any point in your life to help you reach your highest potential. This book has helped me look back at myself and truly ask what I want out of life. It has also helped me see some of my blocks so that now I can get out of my own way to create it. Everyone should read this to reignite their passion for life.

I would like to dedicate this book to a very resilient young woman. You know who you are, and please believe me when I tell you that I am so very proud of you. I cannot begin to express my gratitude and admiration for your beautiful soul. You are a remarkably strong, determined, and powerful being. Despite all of your trauma and turmoil, you continue to carry yourself in a truly kind, respectful, and genuinely loving way. Your unconditional love and empathy for all you meet, along with your curious spirit, fun, loving personality, and unwavering search for growth is what inspires me to wake up each morning and strive for the best in myself. You have brought me hope, reassurance, and guidance when I've needed it the most and I am eternally grateful to you. I hope that this small, but loving gesture honors your goddess spirit in a way that it deserves. You are a magnificent being and wondrous creator. I have so much love for you always.

– **Amanda**

If I'm So Zen, Why is My Hair Falling Out?

IF I'M SO ZEN, WHY IS MY Hair FALLING OUT?

How Anxiety and Past Trauma Manifest in the Physical Body

AMANDA LERA

NEW YORK

LONDON • NASHVILLE • MELBOURNE • VANCOUVER

If I'm So Zen, Why is My Hair Falling Out?

How Anxiety and Past Trauma Manifest in the Physical Body

© 2020 Amanda Lera

Published in New York, New York, by Morgan James Publishing in partnership with Difference Press. Morgan James is a trademark of Morgan James, LLC. www.MorganJamesPublishing.com

ISBN 9781642797985 paperback
ISBN 9781642797992 eBook
ISBN 9781642798005 audio
Library of Congress Control Number: 2019949871

Cover Design Concept: Jennifer Stimson

Cover Design: Megan Dillon   megan@creativeninjadesigns.com

Interior Design: Chris Treccani   www.3dogcreative.net

Editor: Cory Hott

Book Coaching: The Author Incubator

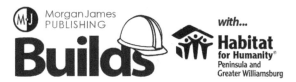

Morgan James is a proud partner of Habitat for Humanity Peninsula and Greater Williamsburg. Partners in building since 2006.

Get involved today! Visit
MorganJamesPublishing.com/giving-back

Table of Contents

Foreword

*A*manda's voice is so universal, so approachable, that it welcomes anyone to read it and connect to at an authentic level. Beautifully constructed and filled with a rich resource of information, Amanda's honest account is highly relatable as well as a valuable tool for anyone who may share these similar circumstances, leading them into a deeper, more loving relationship with themselves. Amanda has captured beautifully the struggles and the challenges that those of service place upon themselves, helping each individual build a stronger connection to themselves while lovingly supporting us all along the way. Very insightful and highly relatable, *If I'm so Zen, Why Is My Hair Falling Out?* spoke to me directly, reminding me to reignite the fires of my own inner love for myself. And whether or not you are losing your hair, or facing the challenges of your body, each and every single one of us can benefit from the words and love within these pages.

Kasia Kaminska

Author of *DRIVERS SEAT...a time traveling manual* and
Co-founder of GiveUpPain.com and the Feeling Path
ILLUMINATED, a Transformational Journey

Chapter 1:

I Got You, Boo

*T*he first time you notice your hair thinning or falling out, it can be jarring. You play it off cool and calm, telling yourself, "There must be a reason for this," but secretly, you are panicking, with a million thoughts running through your head. Is this all part of aging? Is there something seriously wrong with me? Why is this happening to me? What are people going to think? How can I hide this? How can I fix it before anyone notices?

Plenty more thoughts race through your head as the self-doubt sets in. Maybe you've had it wrong this whole time and your diet and exercise haven't actually been right for you. Maybe you are not as calm and composed, mature and professional as everyone portrays you to be. Maybe you don't have the answers and have just been winging it this entire time.

You start to feel like a fraud in every area of your life. You are the strong, independent, intelligent, calming presence that everyone in your life comes to for comfort, reassurance, and advice. If anyone discovers that your hair is falling out or that you have some strange ailment, your credibility is lost. How are you – someone who literally teaches coping mechanisms and calming strategies – being told by a doctor that your hair loss is due to stress? How can you be stressed when you don't feel stressed? There must be another answer, and if you can just get the proper diagnosis, then you can get the cure, fix the issue fast, regrow the hair, and get back to the you that you have convinced yourself you are. No one will ever have to know.

As an instructor or healer, you are expected to have a certain look. If you are leading a "natural" lifestyle, you are expected to be thin and fit, with glowing skin and thick flowing hair. Why would anyone pay to be the student of someone who doesn't look the part? You allow yourself to believe that people will begin to talk, saying things like,

"That teacher clearly doesn't have the answers if she can't even take care of herself." Of course, you feel the pressure to look a certain way – this is your job, but that is what makes this process even more necessary. You cannot teach what you do not know. If you are willing to do the work, the real work – sorry, not a quick fix, but a permanent fix – then you are ready to have that major life change.

If you have seen multiple doctors for second opinions, but received the same answers, tried naturopaths and dermatologists, all to be told that, "It's just stress," but you know it's something more – you must trust that feeling. Nobody knows your body better than you do, and you know instantly when it is not performing the way it usually does. Our bodies have a reason for everything that they do, and it is helping to heal us even when we don't know it. You can spend all the time you want on WebMD or Google searching female bald spots, reasons for hair loss, or sudden hair loss ailments, but let me save you some time because all that will do is send you down a rabbit hole of false self-diagnosis. And trust me, if you aren't stressed now, you will be after that.

There are countless possible medical reasons why people lose their hair, but let's be honest; if you have been properly diagnosed and treated, you aren't reading this book. You are here because you have tried everything else and it either hasn't worked at all or has only worked temporarily. Maybe you spend sleepless nights on WebMD. You went to the doctors, changed your diet, tried smelly creams and awful shampoo treatments, ordered every vitamin and serum on the internet for thick, healthy hair growth, and wasted countless hours on DIY scalp treatments and circulation-stimulating massages. Those are all great, and beneficial to an extent, but if they solved the problem, you wouldn't be here holding this book.

You want to grow your hair back for good this time and you are sick of the temporary fixes. You are sick of dodging humiliating questions like, "OMG! What happened?" or "Gasp! Do you know you have a bald spot right here?" Tired of checking the mirror, covering up with different hairstyles and products, praying it stays in place and keeping from turning your back to anyone? It's exhausting, especially at the gym or on a windy day.

Amber first came to me about her daughter Melissa, asking for recommendations for topical treatments because Melissa's eyebrows were patchy and falling out more each week, to the point where one was almost completely gone. It turned out that Melissa was actually pulling the hairs out herself without even realizing she was doing it. It was a coping mechanism she developed in situations or conversations that made her uncomfortable. Throughout some conversations, I observed the behavior more than once and pointed it out to her. She was completely oblivious to the fact that she was doing it. We all have our nervous ticks or quirks. In the social work field, they are referred to as STIMs, short for stimulations. It is a way that our body calms the mind so that it can focus – similar to a shaky leg under the table, a tapping finger, or chewing a pen during a meeting or class. We all have ways in which our body regulates our emotions, and this was Melissa's.

You may think that simply pointing that out and telling her not to do it was the answer, but like I said, she wasn't aware of it while it was happening, so we needed to find the source of the reaction. Through conversation, observations, activities, surveys, and tests, we were able to determine common triggers and explore them more deeply. Once she was able to identify which situations were making her anxious and why she was then able to catch herself in the act and address the feelings of nervous insecurity in the moment before the reaction to pluck her hairs with her fingers kicked in.

During this time, Melissa's mom, Amber, was losing her eyelashes and not even realizing it until they completely fell out. She didn't identify herself as stressed, mostly because she kept herself too busy to ever really acknowledge any of her own emotions. Amber worked multiple jobs, took on extra projects to help her friends, was raising a family, and running a small business. She did such a great job of telling herself that she was happy, that she pushed down and escaped any thought or emotion that did not support that belief. Her body tried to warn her, but she just kept going until it slowly started manifesting in bigger ways. She neglected to determine the real cause of her hair loss and simply wasn't ready to deal with it at the time. It was a year before she came back after countless failed expensive treatments and was ready to dig deeper to find the solution.

The help is here when you are truly ready and willing to accept it.

You know there is more to your hair loss. You already have the answers inside of you, but perhaps you need some assistance drawing them out or putting them into practice. Your body has been communicating with you, but you just haven't heard the message, and that's okay! That's why I am here – to help source the root cause of the issue and alleviate it for good.

You are not alone. You are stronger than you realize. You are beautiful.

Chapter 2:

My Story

*I*t is going to be alright. I have been where you are, and so have many others. You will save yourself a lot of time, energy, and frustration by committing to the process I have developed. It has provided lasting results for me and my clients, so take a breath – we are in this together.

My hair was my security blanket. It was the source of my confidence. It was a small shield from the outside world. It gave me comfort and a sense of control. To some, that may seem shallow, but it was my identifying quality, and that made me feel safe. I had worn it long my entire life. I was always complimented on how gorgeous it was or how creative my ever-changing styles were. I lived with the belief that if my hair looked good, then I looked good!

Looking back now, it is clear to me that my body tried to communicate the source of my anxiety to me for so long, but I got so good at telling myself I was fine. It was years before I realized that I just wasn't listening. As a child, I was labeled as a hypochondriac. I was curious about everything, but the lack of answers made me fearful. I never knew how to properly express myself, so when questions I asked did not receive responses that satisfied my curiosity, it manifested into a more extreme, paranoid thinking. At the risk of "being dramatic," I learned to keep those things to myself. During moments of panic, I would tell myself I was fine or to just stop, and then would distract myself by pacing and thinking "happier thoughts."

This led to me shutting off my dreams. I remember the exact night it happened. I had been having a reoccurring nightmare but was too embarrassed to talk about it. I prayed to have all my dreams blocked, good or bad. I am sure I still dreamt, but I never remembered them when I woke. As far as I was concerned, there was only darkness while I slept and that was fine by me. Our dreams are one of the ways our body communicates with us. Our subconscious can be uncensored and give great insight into what we are really going through. I shut down that dialogue and it started to spread into my conscious world. I kept myself so busy between a full-time overnight job and a full-time course load in film school. Just like my panicked pacing as a child, I built distractions into my everyday life as an escape from any real feelings. Our true selves have been buried over time by all the emotions we don't want to feel.

My first year of film school, I got paralyzing vertigo. I had gone to the Emergency, saw a number of doctors, spoke with my family doctor, had countless appointments with naturopaths, RMTs, chiropractors, and ENTs. The most I had discovered about my diagnosis was that it was positional. I was on different medications and exercise plans, some of which provided temporary relief, but none were actually preventative. This continued for six months.

This should have been my first indication that there was something out of balance for me and that it was seeking my attention, but I was so good at convincing myself I was fine. I didn't want to use it as an excuse at work or school, so I pushed through and continued to juggle full-time school, full-time work, a relationship, family, an active social life, and sixteen-hour set days for film. During this time, I started to break out in random dry red and white blotches of skin on my legs, and my big toenail had turned yellow. Again, seeking out doctors, naturopaths, and dermatologists only to be put on medications that had no effect. I was told that we all have fungus in the body and sometimes it becomes hyperactive, but will often clear on its own. I kept up with the treatments that I knew were not working because I didn't want to be a bother or appear overly worried about something that shouldn't be a big deal. I didn't want to go back to being seen as a hypochondriac. I was stronger, smarter, and better than that. Or, so I told myself.

In reality, my body had been trying to tell me to slow down and deal with the real issues, but I kept saying I was fine and ignoring it. So, in order to get my attention, it hit me where it hurt the most: my hair! Brennan was the first to notice the missing patch of hair on the back of my scalp. If my hair was what I thought made me beautiful, then how was my boyfriend going to find me attractive and lovable if I lost it? I was humiliated and terrified. I, again, went through my long list of doctors, naturopaths, late nights on Google, Web MD, took every medication, vitamin, used every ointment, shampoo, DIY treatment – literally anything that said it would help regrowth. The medical professionals all chalked it up to stress and the "fungus," which we already knew was running through my body, but I didn't feel stressed, and the fungal treatments weren't working either, so what was I supposed to do?

I convinced myself that I had alopecia. This is when the immune system attacks its own hair follicles, resulting in bald spots. It is reported to be the cause of genetic make-up combined with "other factors" and does not currently have a permanent cure, according to Western medicine. People with alopecia are considered to be a high-risk for other autoimmune diseases, even though it is generally found in otherwise healthy individuals.

I was terrified of what would happen if I lost it all. I convinced myself at one point that it was ringworm (a fungal infection of the scalp and hair shafts) and was worried I was contagious, but there were no signs of either ailment. The skin was perfectly clear, no markings on the scalp or trauma to nearby follicles, but that didn't ease my mind. I thought at least if it could have a diagnosis, then I could heal it faster. I was embarrassed to let anyone find out. I was a yoga teacher and a Reiki practitioner – I couldn't have stress and fungus; what would my clients think of me? I felt like a fraud. I was so careful about the way I styled my hair to hide the perfectly circled patch of hair that was missing. It was completely bald, totally smooth, no baby hair or new hairs in sight. Disgustingly obvious! I taught all my classes with just enough lighting so my students could see me and avoided turning my back to anyone whenever possible. I avoided swimming, which was crazy and awkward. Anyone who knows me knows that I am a total water baby and will swim as long as possible, but the bald spot was even more obvious when my hair was wet. Those were the hardest excuses to come up with. It was easier to say I couldn't go to the beach or barbecue at all than to go and say I can't swim. Like the situation with the vertigo, I assumed that if I made some changes in my life and slowed down to take time for myself, to work on some self-care, then my hair would grow back. And it did! What I didn't realize at the time was that I had eliminated some of the negative situations that I had put myself in and worked on making peace with some past events that caused me pain. But, again, I was only scratching the surface, and although I healed those situations, I did not correct my patterns.

A year later, I was in the exact same performance with different players. I didn't do the work I needed, and my body was there to tell me. That's when the second random chunk of hair fell out, but this time, it was even bigger than the last. All those insecure, embarrassed, humiliating feelings came flooding back. Back to the DIY treatments that I knew weren't working; back to the stupid updos that I hated; back to checking the mirror every time the wind blew, or I moved my head too quickly; back to rocking toques in the summertime. Yup, I was that girl. This was my wake-up call. I knew that if I was to believe that we have the power to make ourselves sick – which I do – then we also have the power to heal ourselves. This was a clear indicator that I had not done the work needed to really heal myself.

A part of me still sees my hair as a security blanket and so my body knows that it is the best way to get my attention. It worked. I was listening. For far too long, I kept telling myself to just keep training and getting certified in new areas of interest that had helped me in some way (yoga, Reiki, Indian head massage, aromatherapy, and other fitness modalities). I insisted that once I attained that next certification, I would then be worthy, successful, authentic, real. I told myself to just keep working forward, which is great for some, but in my case, what I really needed to do was work backward to find the true source of the blocks I had created. What was I protecting myself from and how was it stopping me from leading the life I wanted and deserved? There are times when life gets carried away and

I start to just coast through it again, going with the flow, but I trust my body to bring me back, and it always does.

I have done a lot of self-work since that last patch fell out. I examined my eating habits, sleep schedule, exercise methods, as well as a variety of mental health work, which is where I received the most insight into my hair loss. I began deepening my yoga practice and increasing meditation, sharing my wellness practices, including Reiki, Indian head massage, and aromatherapy. I also worked closely with spiritual counselors who helped me to uncover repressed memories and past traumas so that I could offer the same assistance to my clients. Throughout this book, I will walk you through my step-by-step process in order to allow you the same long-lasting results that I have achieved. While I am thrilled to report that hair loss, for me, has not occurred in years, there is always work to be done. We will never be perfect, but we can make a conscious choice to wake each day striving to be better than we were yesterday. I am so excited and honored to go on this journey with you.

You are a magnificent being capable of anything you put your mind and energy to.

Chapter 3:

Take Back Your Hair

"Healers have tough days. Healers have boundaries.
Healers can say 'No.' Healers can say 'I'm not the healer
for you.' Healers need time to heal."
– Liana Naima

A permanent solution is possible. I'm going to break
things down a bit here for you so that you can use this
book as a tool to optimize your success for regrowth.

Healers and empaths take on a huge responsibility
without even realizing it. I am sure that you are the first

17

one to offer help whenever and to whoever is in need. It isn't even a second thought for you, and yet you do it out of pure love without expecting or accepting anything in return. Do you offer yourself this same love, acceptance, and attention? Would you drop everything when you are in need of yourself? Do you allow yourself to ask for help? Or better yet, do you allow yourself to acknowledge that you, at times, do need help?

All too often, we so easily forget to acknowledge our own needs and feelings. We tell ourselves that we are fine. We tell ourselves that what just happened to us or what we are going through is not a big deal. We tell ourselves that it does not or should not affect our day, or better yet, that we should not *let* it. Let's discuss that for a moment, shall we?

It is true that we are in control of our thoughts and that our thoughts manifest into beliefs and then mirror our reality, but does that mean we should block out certain thoughts? Simply ignoring them or telling the negative thoughts or feelings that they don't have a place here is not resolving anything. I'm sorry to break it to you, but that is part of the problem. You are a beautiful soul and you are justified in your feelings. Your thoughts need the validation they deserve. Please don't misunderstand me here. This is not to say that we should live with these thoughts and let them take over, but we also should not bury them. Acknowledge first that they exist and ask yourself why they chose to come up at this time and in this way? There is a reason for our thinking, and if we do not give our true emotions and thoughts the attention they need, how are we ever supposed to put them at ease? If you break your leg, but you tell yourself that you are fine and that it shouldn't ruin your day, will it just heal itself? Perhaps, in a way, yes, but without proper attention and treatment, the bone will not set properly, the pain will still be there even if you learn to live with it; the leg will never be the same and may be rendered useless.

Our brain is a very powerful part of our body, so when something isn't performing in a way that honors and supports our true selves, why do we simply tell it that it's healed, and expect that to be true? If we allow ourselves the time and space to sit with a less desirable thought and identify where it is coming from while acknowledging that there is value in it, we can then start to heal it and shift our perspective. It is always a matter of perspective. I respect and understand the need or desire to be strong for everybody else, but who do you allow to be strong for you?

Jessie first came to me after noticing thinning on the sides of her head, by her temple. She assumed that it was the cheap box of hair dye that she purchased because she was uncomfortable with her naturally greying hair. She told me that she couldn't afford injections or topical treatments because her husband had just lost his job and she had to support the family. Jessie was an elementary school teacher working in the special education department. During our first conversation, she explained that her mother was battling a very aggressive cancer. Jessie spent all day at work caring for others and came home to do more of the same.

She loved her job, but there were always some difficult days. She didn't want to vent to her husband because she thought she should just be grateful to have a position that supported them while he looked for work. She didn't feel justified saying that she was tired because she needed to be grateful for her health and strength while caring for her mother. She would not allow herself a break because her loved ones were relying on her. She couldn't take a leave from work because that meant putting in for a sub and she felt she had a responsibility to her students. Not wanting to be selfish, she pushed aside her fears about her mother's health in order to remain strong for her mom. She kept a positive attitude for her husband who was struggling to find work, and she even took on extra tutoring hours to cover bills that they had fallen behind on without telling him so he wouldn't feel guilty or emasculated. She kept telling herself that she would take time for herself once things got back on track.

In truth, though, there will always be something or someone that needs your attention. There will always be reasons to delay your self-care or reasons why you feel your emotions don't deserve a platform because someone else is in a worse position and needs your strength. You cannot pour from an empty cup. There is a reason why pilots instruct you to put your breathing mask on before helping others. You need to take care of yourself first before you can properly care for others. We will discuss this further in a later chapter, but for Jessie, we built strategies to help her keep her cup full while pouring from the overflow. I am happy to report that her hair filled back out within a month.

Allow yourself to feel. Allow yourself the time to feel bad if that is where you are. Give gratitude to the bad times that made you strong and allowed you to grow. The good times are your reward for being awesome!

In this book, you will learn my process for identifying the cause of your hair loss and develop a personalized solution to permanently solve your hair loss problem. We will examine the start of the hair loss on a deeper level, while identifying outside contributing factors. I will teach you ways in which our body speaks to us daily, and you will build a stronger relationship with yourself as an individual. I will identify the root of the problem and provide you with some fun, simple, and quick exercises that you can use every day and some useful tools that you can pull from as needed. I will help you to release all that no longer serves you so you can schedule more time for you. I will help you to deepen your understanding of the cause of your own hair loss while teaching you strategies to resolve the issue and provide plenty of tools to take with you to prevent it from happening again despite any obstacles in your way.

No matter what you have gone through or are going through, you will overcome and be better for it and I will hold your hand when you need it and remind you how amazing you are in the event you forget. Allow this moment to be the time you decide to take back control of your body and solve your hair loss problem for good.

You can read this book in order, or pick the chapter that resonates most with you at this time and start there. Trust in your ability. Trust yourself.

I have so much love for you and so much confidence in your potential. I support you completely and am honored to be on this journey with you.

I am grounded in goodness. I am brave. I am valued. I matter.

Chapter 4:

Real World

*"Everyone you meet asks if you have a career,
are married or own a house as if life is some kind of
grocery list, but no one ever asks if you are happy."*
– Heath Ledger

*O*ur daily lives and routines have a deep impact on our perspective, our view of the world, and our view of ourselves. Our body is the truest indicator of what is working for us and what is not. It's our own personal lie detector test. Your immune system is attacking your hair follicles, so what lies or misconceptions have you allowed to be your truth?

It is so easy to get caught up in the hectic routine of our everyday lives. With each generation, our schedules are getting busier and more demanding by the day. There just aren't enough hours in the day. It's no wonder we find ourselves stuck in the same rut year after year. We set beautiful intentions for ourselves, but in the blink of an eye, an entire year has passed us by. Housing prices continue to rise, even when our salary does not, so we are forced to work longer hours or accept higher paying positions out of town, which translates to the same additional hours in our commute time. You feel as though you are living to work instead of the other way around. You find yourself in a less than fulfilling position because it pays the bills, keeps food on the table and allows you some form a social life. Your job, while not ideal, looks good on paper so you can be somewhat proud to tell people what you do when they ask. Even if you know it isn't really what you saw yourself doing or dream to continue doing in the future, it's convenient and you are good at it, so why mess with a good thing, right? What we often fail to acknowledge is that we spend more of our time working than any other activity in our lives. It is only natural that this takes a toll on our mental, physical, and emotional well-being. This is especially true if we are not waking up every morning excited to go to work, being filled with an overwhelming sense of joy and pride in what we do. Burn-out and stress leaves from work are becoming more and more prevalent as the caseload increases. You struggle to find time for the things that really matter to you.

We have unintentionally allowed society to dictate how to live our lives in order to be socially accepted. Have a well-paying job, own a home, start a family, make sure your kids are in a good school, and fill their week with extracurriculars to keep them stimulated and prepare them for their future. Just keep ticking off the itemized list that society has created that tells us we are successful.

Our job is not the only area of comfort holding us back. If you have settled into a routine of complacency just going with the flow, there is a good chance you are simply tolerating many other areas of your life. What is your expected role in your family? Are you the strength, the glue, the one that has it all seemingly together, who everyone turns to in their time of need? The source of strength is often the most neglected. It is understandable to feel isolated.

People often forget to check in with their "strong" friend to see how they are doing or if they are okay. It is easy to assume that you don't need anyone to take care of you because you do such a good job of taking care of yourself. What others fail to realize is that your strength and dependence were developed out of necessity. You have to take care of you because you feel no one else will. You are your most reliable source and that can be heartbreaking and draining, yet you continue to pick yourself up, dust yourself off and keep going. The truth is, you don't have to do this alone. You never ask for help, nor do you accept it, so those around you forget to offer. The belief that this is how life has to be is what has allowed you to undermine your true feelings and ignore signs from the body, which is why your hair loss may have seemed to have appeared out of nowhere. In case you haven't been told yet today, you are truly incredible. Read that again! You are a good person. I know you are having trouble believing that of yourself, but it's true. You are a healer and hero, and it takes great strength to be you.

Unfortunately, our friends are not the only ones who may forget to check in on us. You have done such a good job at being everyone's rock that you have convinced even yourself that you "are fine." This projects into your relations and partnerships. Your partner will give you the love that you believe you deserve. You'll hear that come up again in this book, but it never stops being true. Vulnerability is not a weakness. It is truth, trust, and love. Allow yourself to ask for help. You don't always need to handle it on your own. Being independent is wonderful, but being able to ask for what you need and build support is just as important. Vulnerability is raw and honest and so freeing when you allow yourself to embrace it and free yourself from judgment and embarrassment. Your guard is not serving you; it is telling people how to treat you or mistreat you.

Take a moment here to consider the people you choose to surround yourself with. Are the people in your life nurturing your true self? Are you allowing relations for the sake of companionship or do these people feed your soul? Are you surrounded by people who love and support you while challenging you and opening you up to new possibilities and perspectives? Do they make you a better person or simply feed your ego? Can they grow with you? Build a tribe of like-minded individuals in search of a greater good. Surround yourself with people who inspire you and encourage you to be your best. People you feel safe with and supported by and who see you and appreciate you for the amazing and generous being that you are.

It is no coincidence that we use the word "growth" in both the physical and metaphysical state. There is a study where two of the same species of plants are placed on opposite sides of a room. One is bullied verbally throughout the day, while the other is complimented. After the trial, the plant that was complimented, flourished and grew; its roots were strong, and it reproduced other healthy plants. The plant that was bullied did not grow as tall; its leaves and stems withered, and its seeds were unable to reproduce. While the study is shedding light on bullying, its results hold true in other factors. If you do not feel valued, appreciated, or understood in your job, relationships, friendships, home or social life, your mental and physical health becomes stunted over time. Hair loss is a clear indication of imbalance.

Stop making excuses for the relationships that you know no longer serve you, but are familiar, comfortable, or you feel guilty letting go of. Not everyone you meet is meant to be in your life forever. Some people come into your life at a specific time to help you grow to the next phase of your life, and once they have served their purpose, they are meant to move on. Clinging to relations that keep you stuck stunt your growth and project a stagnant energy outward that manifests inward. The universe will continue to provide us with what we ask it for. If you are convinced that this is the best you can do, then that is the best you will do, and the universe will keep providing you with situations that prove or support those beliefs. Step out of the lies that you are telling yourself and strive from something more. You deserve better.

Your body is the first and truest indicator of a complication or imbalance in your life. When we learn to listen to and work with it, we are able to solve and prevent much of what ails us.

I am compassionate. I am bold. I am boundless.

Chapter 5:

Not Again

*I*n this chapter, we will uncover the root cause of your hair loss and identify if you are ready to embrace this process fully in order to solve it for good and take back your hair. It is not an overnight fix. It is easy to think that the journey is complete when you are only halfway. There is real work to be done but I assure you, if you are open and ready, it will be life-changing.

As you begin to heal the surface trauma – the situations that you can readily identify, like an argument or loss of some kind – you will experience a strong sense of relief and clarity. You will likely assume that you have cleared your block – the feelings that have kept you stuck – and have finally let go. That is partly accurate and you may even notice regrowth at this point, but the reality is that your reaction to each trauma that you experience in your adult life is somehow linked to an event or experience we had as a child, so in order to fully free ourselves from its grasp and prevent the hair from just falling out again in a few months, we must dig much deeper.

Situations resonate with us so deeply based on the preconceived notions that we developed in our earlier years. Now, the tricky part here is that the survival instinct is still very strong within us, whether we are attuned to it or not. Our minds have a way of protecting us from emotions that we don't want to feel and, in turn, can block out the memory of events that caused us pain as children. We may not even remember that it happened until something triggers the memory and then, in an instant, we are whisked back into the moment as if it is happening all over. You can see the entire scenario so clearly and vividly, and may even be able to remember specific feelings, colors, scents or sounds.

Our mind is a powerful partner. Digging through the childhood events or roots of the trauma can be a very painful and difficult process. Many individuals are content clearing the surface and feeling that initial sense of relief and then carrying on exactly as they were but feeling slightly more accomplished and clear. That sense of clarity and calm will only last for so long and the body will start to indicate a deeper healing that needs to be addressed.

The most common way that I have seen this manifest in my clients is through migraines and panic attacks. The most subtle thought or feeling can trigger a full-blown attack as if from nowhere, but we know by now that the body reacts for a reason. It is trying to get a message across and the more we ignore it, the louder it has to be. Unfortunately, instead of identifying that there must be deeper healing to be done, most people will think that since they already "did the work" and felt better, it must be something more serious, that there must be something terribly wrong with them. The insecurities and self-judgment pile up more and more, and the feeling of failure becomes overwhelming.

Have you ever noticed that when one thing goes wrong, it feels as though there is a domino effect and one by one, everything seems to fall apart all at once? This is when the body steps in yet again to get our attention. If you aren't listening to the migraine, maybe the panic attack will get your attention. No? Okay, how about a sore throat? Still nothing? Well vertigo is bound to slow you down and if that doesn't work, it gets louder and louder until it stops you dead in your track and forces reflection and change.

For me, it was my security blanket – my hair. The first patch fell out and I vowed to do whatever it took to grow it back before anyone noticed or started asking questions. I did the work, made improvements, felt relief and the hair came back but I had only scratched the surface. I had not healed the deeper issues. As a result, a year later I found myself in the same cycle and routine but with different people and positions. That is when the second chunk fell out and was twice the size of the first one, and next to impossible to hide. I was absolutely humiliated. I was convinced that I had done everything wrong and that everything I had believed to be true must have been false. The reality was that I just had not gone back far enough into my past to identify earlier traumas that I was unknowingly carrying with me. This is what was preventing me from bringing about real healing and permanent change. I had a lot more work to do and it wasn't always easy or enjoyable, but it was necessary and so freeing. A big part of it was apologizing to myself for allowing treatment from others that I did not deserve.

I allowed others to tell me when my feelings were real. I needed my parents or siblings to validate my fears as a child. If I didn't get the validation I sought, I started to bury the fears and emotions that didn't get me the reactions I wanted from others. I carried this through much of my life, never feeling validated in my opinions or emotions. I kept them to myself. More often, I kept them from myself. I convinced myself that I had overcome my fears, but in reality, I just wasn't allowing myself to think about anything that scared me. This had a greater ripple effect than I had realized. I started hiding other negative emotions from myself. I told myself that I was overreacting if I ever felt hurt or anger towards others. I was afraid to express grief or sadness because I feared that it would be portrayed as weakness. I had convinced myself that I was not worthy of the emotion and taught myself to bury it before expressing it.

I had to apologize to myself for moving on before letting go, for keeping myself stuck and for doubting my strength and potential. I apologized for needing acceptance and validation from others over myself as if they were more important or of higher worth.

From such a young age, we are taught to hold on, and we carry that throughout our lives. Hold on to your mother's hand. Hold on to your favorite toys. Hold on to your friendships. Hold on to your job. Hold on to your partner. Hold on, hold on, hold on. It is no wonder that the concept of letting go is so terrifying and misconceived with a loss of control or loss of self. It is this fear that keeps us stuck – stuck in jobs, relations, beliefs, and thoughts that do not serve us. We live in this fear – fear of the inevitable, fear of loss, fear of failure, fear of success or greatness.

What would it mean to you to overcome this fear? What would your life look like? How might you be different? How might the world be different?

I met Mya after her graduating year of university. She had returned to school as a mature student in her early thirties. Mya sunk her life savings into her studies and finished at the top of her class. She dreamed of opening her own business but put her plans on hold after a pipe burst in her bathroom. She was already struggling to keep up with her mortgage payment while juggling car payments and student loans. She was working two jobs just make ends meet and had to pick up and extra shift for three weeks to cover the cost of the plumber. It was at this time that she noticed her hair thinning. The parts in her hair were more pronounced and her hair felt brittle.

Whenever we discussed her plans for the business, Mya would light up with excitement and her ideas would flow so naturally. She appeared so clear and confident on our calls but when I would ask about her progress, there was always a reason why that week was too busy to start building the business. I was starting to notice this pattern throughout other areas of her life. She seemed to be clear on what success looked like for her but was always waiting for something else to happen before she could achieve her goals. "Once the bathroom is fixed, I will be able to focus." "I have to work extra shifts this week to cover my bills but next month my schedule won't be as crazy" "I just need to save a bit more money so maybe I can start next year"

She talked about her business plans with family, friends and coworkers. She had the support and validation from those around her, but she continued to put up these blocks in her own mind. Mya was terrified of her own success, not because of the time or amount of work that would go into it, Mya was used to working long hours. She was afraid that she wasn't good enough to run her own business. She compared herself to others in the field and believed that if she was able to compete, that it somehow meant that she was tricking her clients into thinking that she actually had something to offer. The reality is that she did have something of value to offer but was consumed with self-doubt and feelings of inadequacy. She knew starting a business was a huge time commitment and she told herself that she just didn't have the time. She didn't want to let her current bosses or coworkers down by taking time off or reducing her hours and what about the financial investment? A business is expensive, and she did not have extra funding. She couldn't ask for help with finances. What if she failed? What if she was never able to pay back the money? She feared being a disappointment in the eyes of her family.

Mya didn't realize it at the time, but these insecurities were manifesting in outside barriers that allowed her excuses to keep putting off her dreams. She wasn't truly fulfilled in her life. She felt undervalued and overlooked. A part of her knew that she was destined for more, but she was stuck, and it started to show in her hair. Through deeper conversation and guided practices, I was able to help Mya identify the fears that were holding her back. We developed a personalized schedule to aid in productivity with simple, achievable daily steps to reach a weekly goal. She noticed an improvement in the texture and shine of her hair in the first two weeks. Within three months, her hair was fuller, the parts were smaller, and she had a business plan and strategy for her launch. Mya is now her own boss.

A dream written down with a date becomes a goal. A goal broken down into steps becomes a plan. A plan backed by action becomes reality!

I am the source of my own healing. I am wise. I am calm. I am good.

Chapter 6:

What Lies Beneath

We tend to let our job status or relationships identify who we are. In this chapter, I want to explore the individual you – just you; no title or tie to family, friendship, or partner.

Let's get to know you a little better. The real you, not the you whom others see or whom you are when there is someone watching, but the real, raw, authentic, unapologetically you. I am referring to the guilty-pleasure you. The person you allow yourself to be when no one else is around. If you had an entire day to yourself – no to-do list and no one home but you – how would you spend your time? I am sure if someone called and said, "Hey what are you up to?" You would reply with a list of things you think you should be doing, like cleaning the house, meditating, reading a book, watching an inspirational documentary, working out, or finishing a project. What are you actually doing? What mind-numbing show are you actually watching? Did you really meditate or work out, or was the acknowledgment of saying your intention aloud enough?

Don't be shy, we've all done it. We build these personas for ourselves, but the best way to get to know the real you is to identify who you are when no one else is watching or needing anything from you. We spend so much of our lives surrounded by others, at work, in social settings, and with family. Even when these interactions are positive experiences and we are willing participants, a part of ourselves is slightly compromised. Who are you outside of the colleague, partner, or friend? Who are you when it is just you? What gets you excited? It is so easy to overlook the sacrifices or compromises that we make on a daily basis, especially if they are positive, like settling on Mexican takeout when one partner wants pizza and the other wants Chinese. The important part is enjoying a meal together, so you are willing to overlook your pizza craving.

Every interaction throughout our day is some level of compromise from one person or the other. While that is beautiful and necessary in healthy relationships, it can be so easy to lose sight of ourselves. Your world is built around "we" and "us" and you can forget who the "I" is. Then when the relationship ends, you are left wondering who you are on our own as an individual, outside of the partnership. Through no fault of our partners, we, as nurturers, are just willing to structure our lives to fit others. Over time, this can take quite a toll, as the people in our lives come to expect a certain level of compromise, and if you are unable to ask for the same in return or just expect the same in return, you will find yourself drained and frustrated with a confused partner who doesn't quite understand what has changed or why. It is in these moments when we are compromising the honor of ourselves that our bodies become reactive, and we will notice subtle changes. These reactions appear on the outer body, like our hair, as an indicator of a greater imbalance within the body.

For example, say there is an event that you read about and are really interested in going to, but your partner has a football game that day and has asked you to come. You go to support your partner and think nothing of it at the time. Another event will come up, but other commitments always seem to arise, and you feel like you are missing out on more and more of what you want in order to appease those around you. You tell yourself that it isn't a big deal and that it isn't being forced on you; you have chosen it, so you are fine. Over time, resentment starts to build and eventually you are feeling like your relationships are one-sided, with you putting in all the work and not receiving it in return. You are left feeling unsupported, underappreciated, and taken for granted. Sound familiar? It happens so gradually, but you have been telling people how to treat you and then question how it got this far.

When I met Clara, she was concerned about her hair thinning on the top front region of her head. At the time, she had been with her partner Paul for two years. She really loved him and truly enjoyed their time together. He had a very busy schedule and was raising two children, but she felt their relationship was strong. Clara happily accompanied him to his children's sporting events and recitals, Paul's football games, family functions, and countless other social commitments. Their weekends were always full. She willingly rearranged her schedule to fit his, not because he asked her to, but because she wanted to be with him and knew it made him happy to have her company. They spent plenty of time together, but it was always fulfilling other commitments. They did not often have quality time together where it was just the two of them.

After two years, Clara started to feel like she was constantly compromising and missing out on her interests in order to accompany Paul to his. She felt like she was completely submerged in his world, but he was not really a part of hers. Clara could sense herself becoming more defensive, distant, and angry with Paul and he didn't seem to understand why. She decided that she had to either miss the event that she was interested in or go alone because his schedule was usually so packed. She thought it was more important to support him, but felt as though she were losing a part of her own identity. She never actually had this conversation with Paul. She feared telling him because she thought she would lose him. She worried she was being selfish, but not addressing it led to more unresolved arguments and more noticeable hair loss.

Paul had no idea that she was feeling this way because she never voiced her needs, but he could sense that something had changed within their relationship in a negative way. It was causing him stress and anxiety, but he did not know how to address it either. He feared being vulnerable because he saw it as a weakness. I worked with them over the course of two months to break some old habits and open the lines of communication. Clara was finally able to voice her own needs in order to build a stronger, more supportive relationship with her partner and others in her life. This voice was the remedy to her regrowth.

Allow yourself to ask for what you need without feeling guilty or embarrassed. Vulnerability is honest and courageous. It can be scary to be vulnerable, even around those we love the most, but it is a sign of love, trust, and security. If there is something you really want to do, but it doesn't fit into your current schedule, find the next available time and don't be afraid to express to your partner, why this event is so significant to you.

It will not always work out that your friend or partner is available or even interested in everything you are, and that's okay. It's actually great. It doesn't mean you need to miss out. It means that you get to experience it on your own. Going out solo may seem lame or pathetic to most, but it is actually so liberating. You will strengthen your independence, confidence, and connection with self. It is freeing to be able to do an activity you enjoy and be fully submerged in it mentally without feeling like you are dragging someone with you or wondering if they are having a good time. It will feel a little uncomfortable at first, but it is like living alone. It's scary the first time you do it, but then you start to wonder how you ever shared your space. This knowledge and self-awareness teaches you what you need in a partner or roommate in order to feel right sharing your space again.

Learning to enjoy your own company is so important. It allows you to identify who you are and what you really want. When you enjoy time with yourself, you allow yourself to be more selective in the relationships you choose, making those interactions and relations so much deeper, more intimate, and long-lasting. We operate with the illusion of freedom, but we rarely achieve it.

When we aren't surrounding ourselves with others, we have technology to fill the silence, music, shows, funny videos, or posts from friends. When was the last time you were out to dinner and the person you were dining with got up to use the bathroom and you did not pull out your phone? We can't even be alone with ourselves for five minutes. We have trained ourselves to need constant stimulation, but we have also engrained in our subconscious that we are being watched and judged as we are just sitting there with nothing to do.

We are projecting our insecurities through our inability to be alone with ourselves. We have allowed silence to be our greatest fear. All of our answers are in that silence.

Our deepest thoughts, desires, interests, perceptions, judgments, creative bursts, pleasures and pains all come to surface in the silence and we have allowed that to be so frightening that we don't let ourselves enjoy it or learn from it. Next time you are in line for coffee, avoid the temptation to look down at your phone, and just observe. Enjoy one whole minute of uninterrupted time with you and let the coffee be your reward. It gets easier over time and I promise that you are going to start to crave alone time. You share all your own interests. You are your own best friend. When you love you, your project love and show others how to love you in the way you truly deserve. You never have to settle for a companion for the sake of company or worry about missed opportunities because you are enough.

When we devote more time to identifying who we are as an individual, we uncover more truths about our personality, interests, needs, and desires. We become more in-tune with what we want and what we are willing to give in return. This knowledge allows us the ability to build more stable and longer lasting relationships with people deserving of our love and attention. Empower yourself by sharing your life with those who honor and feed your soul.

I am worthy. I am glorified. I am truth.

Chapter 7:

Body Talk

*L*isten to your body when it whispers so you don't have to hear it scream.

Our body has so many ways of trying to communicate with us. Let's start with the basics. Take it down to the simple foundation: the breath. The breath is so easily overlooked and yet the root and life of all that we do. The breath, if you are able to identify and listen to it, will be the first indicator of the state of your physical and mental health. Think about it: What happens to our breath when we are scared? It quickens, perhaps even shortens, then our hearts race and our body temperature rises; we become lightheaded or short of breath, and panic sets in. On the flip side, what happens to our breath when we are calm? Our breathing is smoother, deeper, our body cools and stills. We feel relaxed. I can feel the change in my body just as I write these words. Our breath is a very powerful tool and yet we take it for granted.

The first thing that I teach in all of my yoga and fitness programs, regardless of the level, is the breath. Our breath can alert us to our true emotional state and can also indicate minor to severe health issues. Controlling our breathing is the first step in taking control of our bodies, our actions, and our health. Thirty seconds of simply counting the breaths as they enter and exit your body can completely alter your mood and clear your thoughts. It calms us, and being calm allows your mind to find solutions. Calmness is a state of trust. Instead of overthinking and overreacting, allow yourself to surrender just for the moment and receive guidance for the things that aren't making sense. Aside from the physical benefits this will create in the body – lower blood pressure, lower heart rate and cortisol (stress response), promote relaxation and strengthen the diaphragm – it will also provide you with the clarity to answer questions you didn't even know you had. Those "ah-ha" moments are made in silent reflection.

Have you ever been working so diligently on a work assignment or paper that you get stuck on how to word your next phrase or what else to include? You sit there staring at the screen and when you finally decide to take a break, you get up to get a coffee and it hits you. The answer is so clear and so simple. What you failed to realize is that moment that you allowed yourself the break, you likely had a sense of relief and let out an extended breath. You gave yourself that moment of clarity and perhaps unintentional trust that the answer would come if you just took a moment. The body responded.

The majority of us have conditioned our bodies to reverse breathe, which leads to a long list of health problems by itself. Reverse breathing is very common, especially in us ladies, as society tells us to appear slim and trim, yet busty. We have a tendency to suck our bellies in and puff our chests out, and when we can't hold it in any longer, we exhale and let it all out. If this sounds familiar, you are a reverse breather.

The body is meant to expand on the inhale, taking in all the fresh oxygen and filling the body. Picture your torso like a balloon. When we inhale, we want to fill that balloon so our stomach and sides should expand outward and our chest should fill and rise. Then on the exhale, think about squeezing every last bit of air out of that balloon as your stomach, sides, and chest compress to release toxins. This allows our diaphragm to operate the way it is intended.

Now the real magic and beauty of our bodies is that, despite the years spent conditioning and training our bodies to reverse breathe, the moment we fall asleep, the body takes over and corrects this for us. Our body is truly amazing and will take all the twisted thinking and social norms we throw at it throughout the day and just correct it. Our body is constantly working to try to reverse the damage we do to it on a daily basis. All we have to do is learn to listen.

Connecting to nature can be a beautiful way of connecting to the breath. Breathing exercises in themselves can be anxiety-inducing for someone who is not used to the practice. Going out for a walk or light jog can help you to identify changes in the breath based on the weather or your pace, and gauge how your thoughts and feelings change (good or bad) in those moments. The earth emits negative ions, which have a laundry list of healing benefits (check out the back of the book or contact me for more detail on this), so whenever possible, walk barefoot in nature or on the grass in your backyard. Simply place one hand on your chest and breathe. Bask in the security, comfort, and positive energy that the ground has to offer.

Like our breath, our body has countless ways of trying to talk to us. It may start off small, with a cramp, a stomachache, or a headache. If ignored, it may manifest into something more intense, like a migraine, nausea, ulcer, fungal infection; the list goes on and on. Have you ever heard someone say, "Stop stressing. You're going to give yourself an ulcer," or, "an aneurysm," or, "cancer?" I've said these things to people myself because I believe that the brain is a very powerful organ. I honestly believe that we have the power to make ourselves sick. The wonderful thing about that is, if you believe this like I do, then that means we also have the power to heal ourselves in many situations.

Often times, all we have to do is identify the cause. I have learned, over time, that if I have a scratchy sore throat and no other cold symptoms – which is often the case – it is because there is a situation that I have not addressed. It can be something simple, like a disagreement with a family member, but if I don't address it in the moment, I will wake the next day with a sore throat and it will not go away until I resolve the matter in a way that honors me. Sometimes it is as easy as acknowledging that the interaction bothered me and simply validating myself by saying it out loud. Other times, I will need to write it out in order to get it out of my head, and if it still lingers, then I know I have to address that person and speak my truth. Often times, we just ignore these subtle warnings from the body, but it is alerting us that something is out of balance. We medicate out of convenience because it is what we know, but it just manifests. Eventually, the body will come up with new and more alarming ways of getting its point across. For me, it was vertigo and then, when that wasn't enough, my hair started to fall out.

Prince Ea is an American spoken word artist, poet, and filmmaker. He has a very powerful video on how our thoughts affect our mental health. In it, he states, "You wouldn't eat a rotten tomato because it would make you sick and yet we accept all these poisonous thoughts into our head and then wonder why they have the same effect." No, you may not throw up, but you will definitely give yourself aches and pains that present themselves physically and lead to much more serious mental ailments, like anxiety or depression. Too often, our thoughts and feelings are suppressed or invalidated. In our culture, we are never taught the importance of healing. We are taught only to survive. We have not been taught how to identify and heal our past trauma or mental health struggles. We are taught to ignore it, bury our "weakness" and survive. There is a flaw in that system. If we don't heal, we don't grow. We don't better ourselves. We relive the same pain, and at the point, survival is less enticing.

When we break our symptoms and triggers down, the answers are often clear. This means not only acknowledging the hurt, but addressing it. Our true selves have been buried over time under all the emotion we don't want to feel.

Often times, our symptoms can be traced back to a very specific event. If we are willing to look closer and dig a little deeper, we can identify it and resolve it. Take, for instance, the wasp story. A man is walking through the park and is stung by a wasp. He lets out a surprised yell, but brushes it off and continues on his way. Once home, his arm is quite sore. When he goes to clean it, he notices that it is swollen. He puts some ointment on and carries on about his day. Later that night, as he is walking into a local pub, he runs into an old friend that excitedly grabs him by the arm, right above his swollen elbow yelling, "Hey buddy, good to see you." The friend obviously had no idea what happened earlier or that the man was in pain, and certainly did not mean any harm. The man jumped back, cursing at the friend initially, but then takes a moment to explain what happened and apologizes.

The point of the story is that we are all walking around with these underlining injuries. Often, we don't even realize that they bothered us in the first place, or maybe we just never got the opportunity to resolve them, so we forget about it until somewhere down the road, someone hits that trigger and now becomes the source of your misplaced anger or emotional baggage. The man never gave a second thought to the wasp that stung him. It seemed so insignificant at the time but later proved to be a bigger issue.

You will hear me say this again and again: Your body is talking to you. All you have to do to find the answers is listen. When your body eats something it cannot handle, you get sick; if it receives a medical treatment that is too much for it, your body rejects it; yet when we are dealing with trauma or repressed emotions, our body responds the same way; we choose not to acknowledge or believe it to be true. Trust that your body is looking out for you. It is working to heal you even when you are fighting against it. Become its ally. Partnering the body with the mind will allow you to overcome.

I am certain. I am supported. I am a powerful creator.

Chapter 8:

Taking a Selfish

*I*n this chapter, I am giving you permission to say "no" every once in a while. I am sure you've never tried it, but I assure you, it feels great. We often feel obligated to say "yes" to plans or a request to help someone move, et cetera, simply because we have been asked. Even if our schedule is crazy and we are exhausted and desperately want a bath and early night, we still say yes. It will be fun, so why pass up the opportunity to see a friend? So and so really needs my help. It is impolite to turn down an invitation. Sound familiar?

Do not ever underestimate the power and necessity of "taking a selfish." That word has so much negativity attached to it, but does it have to? Think about it; In chapter 3, I mentioned that we would come back to the metaphor that you cannot pour from an empty cup. That is, of course, true but you also should not be required to pour from a full cup because you will again start to give more than you can and deplete your own resources and energy. Instead, what I am going to suggest to you is to keep yourself constantly flowing throughout your day. Honor yourself in a way that not only fills your cup, but overflows it, and then pour from your overflow. Allow yourself to stay full and give away all the extra that flows through you.

Reiki is a beautiful example of this practice because it is the belief that we as practitioners are simply a conduit for the universe's energy. It flows through us and into whoever is receiving it. This protects our energy from being drained by those we come in contact with, but also allows us to receive the energy as we share it with others.

It may seem selfish or inconsiderate to look after yourself first, but if you are not properly taken care of, then how can you ever properly care for anyone else without eventually burning out? Allow yourself a "selfish" and let's make that a positive thing. Take time in your day, even if it is just ten minutes, and do something that truly honors you. Step outside for some air, take a bath, listen to your favorite song, walk a flight of stairs, do some pushups – anything that allows you to completely shut out the world. No phones, no kids, no work for those brief periods of time, and do one thing that makes you smile and feel good about yourself. Allow yourself as many of these little breaks as you need throughout the day, but at least try to get one in each day and remind yourself that the mile-long to-do list you are stepping away from will still be there when you return, but you will return more prepared to take it on. A mere thirty seconds of listening to the breath as it flows in and out of the body can do so much to clear your thoughts, boost your memory and creativity, calm your nerves, lower your blood pressure, and boost your mood. We all have thirty seconds. Start small and work your way up. Ideally giving yourself at least an hour every day to do something just for you.

It is empowering and will make such a difference in the way you carry yourself and conduct yourself in your interactions with others. You will notice subtle positive changes immediately. Try, if you can, not to allow yourself to get caught up in the guilt of "taking a selfish." Remember, it's a good thing. Clear your mind again by

Often the hardest part is saying, "No," which is why I suggest taking time away from distractions. There are so many times when we intend to do something for ourselves or promise ourselves that after we do this, we will have time for that, but the time for that never comes because we get a call, a text, or asked for a favor, and we feel the need to say yes. We allow ourselves to feel obligated to go out simply because someone asked us to, even if we aren't particularly interested. We feel obligated to complete a task because "it's just better if I do it myself." We never ask for help, but always offer it. It is nice to feel needed and it also gives us an excuse not to get things done because something else came up. Something else will always come up. Learn to embrace the relief and power of "no." It's okay. It doesn't have to be a bad thing or an insult if it is what you need. You don't have to concoct some long-winded excuse. A simple, "I can't tonight," is enough. Let it be enough and if it makes you feel better, reschedule for another more convenient time for you.

We get so caught up in the hustle and bustle of life that when we do have a few moments in our day, we often think, "I must be forgetting something," as if there is something wrong with not constantly being busy. This was a real struggle for me. I worked full-time while juggling school full-time, running around helping others in my spare time and trying to get a business off the ground. When I had thirty minutes to eat a meal or sit on the couch, I actually thought I was being unproductive and felt really bad about myself like there was something more I should be doing. I had a friend teach me to crochet just so I could sit and watch a full episode of a TV show while still feeling like I was being useful. No wonder I lost my hair, right?

But the question is, "Why?" Why did I need to be that busy? Why was I allowing myself to be so negative if I ever stopped? Why couldn't I just be with me, without a distraction? I didn't know who I was and staying busy helped me feel relevant, useful, worthy, loveable, and needed. Staying busy helped me avoid truths about myself that I did not like. The poor decisions that I had made in my past that I was not proud of. It was an escape, but as we now know, buried emotions turn up somewhere in the physical body, like our hair.

Why is taking a selfish so hard? It isn't really because of the negative ties to the word. It is because we are so afraid to be alone with ourselves, alone with our own thoughts. Ask yourself, "Why?" What are you hiding from? What are you running away from? What is it that you are not allowing yourself to feel? You know the answer, but are you willing to give it the justification and validation it deserves? Start a dialogue with yourself and your thoughts, but talk to yourself the way you talk to someone you love. There's a saying that if we fix our thoughts, then our problems fix themselves, but we first have to identify the source of our thoughts and then apologize to ourselves for accepting what we did not deserve.

Take time for you and release yourself from the guilt of doing so. You will thrive and you will be so much better for those around you. Pour from your overflow!

I am in a safe space. I am confident. I am abundant.

Chapter 9:

Letting Go

The first step to letting go of our trauma is to first acknowledge that there is trauma. It has been a long and sometimes painful road to acknowledging my own trauma. I spent years blissfully unaware and did not allow myself to believe that anything bad had ever happened to me. I was always told what a fun, happy, easy-going, free-spirited individual I was. It must be wonderful to be me. I believed it to be true and would not allow myself to be anything but that perception of myself. Despite anything that happened, I always thought, "I don't have it bad. I am definitely not a victim. There are way worse things that people go through and far worse things happening around the world every day." While that is true, it did not change the fact that things were happening in my life that were leaving scars. I allowed myself to undermine my hardships and my pain. I trained myself to believe that if it isn't "that bad," then it didn't need acknowledgment or healing. That created so many blocks for me and really stunted my growth.

As we downsize our grief or pain, we make it okay for others to do the same. We get stuck in this cycle of telling ourselves that we haven't experienced anything "that bad." We have never overcome any great obstacle. In this way, we completely overlook the strength and courage that it took to survive these traumas and move past them. We allow ourselves to believe that what we have just achieved is nothing. We are not an inspiration in any way. We have no story to tell or message to share. That simply isn't true. We are not the mediocre, average Joes that we portray ourselves to be. You may call it modesty, but what you are really doing is extinguishing your flame. You are turning off your own light and blocking others from the warmth in the process. In doing so, you are telling yourself that you are not special, you have nothing to offer, you are just doing what anyone else in your position would do, but that is not the case. Words are energy. Be gentle and kind in the way you use them, especially with yourself. That energy will be projected out into the world and returned back to you.

You did not allow your trauma to break you. You remained strong for everyone around you. Your strength is admirable, and you deserve the healing you so freely and willingly share with others. You deserve the support and unconditional love that you dish out without a second thought. You deserve to be cared for the way you so generously care for others. Your trauma exists inside of you, but it does not define who you are, and it does not deserve to live inside of you. It served its purpose in your life the second you acknowledged how you have grown from it. Now, you are free to release it. Allow yourself the justification and validation you give others.

When I was seventeen, a friend and coworker of mine was murdered in a home invasion. I had experienced a lot of death in my life by that time, but never had someone been taken from me in that way. Most of the death I experienced was from natural causes, aside from my uncle who had taken his own life, but I had managed to justify that in my head as his choice. When my friend was murdered, I had no idea how to process it. My friends and family tried to be supportive, but I was so confused and angry that I didn't know what I needed to heal.

I got so wrapped up in the case, keeping every newspaper clipping, and attending every hearing. I guess I thought that if his killer was proven guilty, then it would somehow make it okay, or at least tolerable. The guilty parties showed no remorse and I sat there every day watching how it tore my friend's family apart.

I spent so many nights locked away in my room because I wasn't able to fake that happy little girl smile for everyone. I felt so guilty about the fact that my friends and family were so worried about me. I couldn't allow myself to really grieve my friend or process my pain because I was so consumed with the thought that I was letting people down by not being perfect and happy and letting it all roll off my shoulder like the fun-loving, passive, easy-going girl that I told myself I was supposed to be. It was a real struggle, and looking back, there were more times than I can count that I put that level of pressure on myself. Seems kind of silly now to even question why my hair is was falling out, right?

If we cannot validate our emotions, how are we to understand the root of our problem in order to fully heal and release? Eventually, our body steps in to alert us to the blocks we have been avoiding. Trust that your body is talking to you out of love. It works overtime to heal us, but it needs the help and partnership of the mind.

There are going to be times where you realize something is sitting with you that you may not have identified as bothering you in the moment. I find this happens most at bedtime. It is one of the rare moments when we allow ourselves to be alone in silence. If you have ever experienced insomnia or racing thoughts, you know exactly what I'm talking about. Maybe you have used a noise machine or music to help you sleep. Perhaps you are someone who falls asleep to the TV, and for the most part, that helps. Then there are the nights where no amount of distraction can quiet the mind.

These are the nights when I am going to challenge you to pay attention. Make a mental note of your breathing during this time. Take out a note pad – and you don't have to be neat about this – but scribble down all the thoughts that are racing through your head. Single keywords or bullet point form is fine as long as it makes sense to you. Keep up with your thoughts as best you can and get it all out on paper. You may even need to say it out loud as you write. Giving these thoughts a platform or physical presence can be liberating and validating. Often times, it is enough simply to get the thoughts out of your head, even if you do nothing with it after.

You may choose to immediately rip it up and discard it. You could burn it and release it, or you may want to leave it on your nightstand. I keep a scrap piece of paper and pen on my night stand and often scribble down notes to release before laying down for a restful sleep. These thoughts are in your head for a reason. Get them out and give them a temporary place to live outside of your mind while you get some sleep, again making a mental note of how your breathing changed, if at all, after this.

Then, in the morning, or when you have a minute to yourself, go back to your scribble pad and read each one out loud. Do you have a noticeable physical sensation or reaction to anything on that page? A tingle, a cramp or pain, twitch in the eye? Does your stomach flip or heart sink? That is your guide, your source, your gut, your navigator. Whatever you want to call it, that is your body's natural instinct telling you that there is something there you need to address. Maybe it is as simple as admitting it to yourself that something is bothering you or feels incomplete and needs closure or resolve. You will learn what feels right and what you need for yourself in order to achieve that closure in a way that honors you so that you can release it for good. I can help you with this. I have offered you a few strategies for this in the next chapter. You will know it is right when you feel at ease. This may mean speaking to someone directly or drafting an email to that person, even if you never actually send it.

Welcome whatever emotion arises. Avoid the need or impulse to push it down and tell yourself you are overreacting or insisting that you are fine and asking yourself to calm down. Try to sit with this emotion instead. Allow yourself to feel sad, hurt, or fearful. Sit with the feeling and see if it can pass over instead of being pushed down. They are just thoughts that we are giving power to. Take back your power. Identify what it is that is triggering the response. What is it that you really need? Why is it having this effect on you and what would it look like to resolve it?

You know you have honored your true self when you feel peace with thoughts or situations where there was once tension.

Holding on to the past does not aid or honor you. We cannot change the past, but we can certainly learn from it. Take the lessons with you, but release the hurt, guilt, resentment, or anger. Move forward stronger and wiser for having survived what you have, and take pride and comfort in knowing that the knowledge you have gained will help you to build a more peaceful future. When we protect the lesson and release the trauma, we prevent history from repeating.

You survived the abuse. You are going to survive the recovery.

I am free. I am safe. I am relief. I am peace.

Chapter 10:

Tool Box

*Y*ay! Welcome to the fun stuff. This chapter is full of great activities and practices to strengthen the connection to your true self so you can really start to enjoy your own company.

Have fun with it.

Start off with a morning ritual. It doesn't have to be anything strenuous or time-consuming. You can check out my five-minute morning yoga bed routine to get your day started on the right foot before you even leave your cozy, warm bed. Morning rituals are the easiest way to retrain your brain because it sets the tone for your entire day. If yoga isn't for you, try a journal. Wake up and write the first thing that comes to mind that you are grateful for and then set an intention for your day – short and simple, but it activates your brain and starts your day with love and positivity. You could take a quick five- to ten-minute walk around your block for a burst of fresh air and inspiration to start your morning, or change it up each day based on your mood. The idea is to accomplish something in the time it takes for you to brew your morning coffee. Banging one accomplishment out right at the start of your day boosts your mood, attitude, and productivity for the rest of the day.

I took a training course recently with Ben Greenfield and he highlighted the benefits of low-dose, high-effective body movements. I love the kind of workouts where you don't feel like you are working out, but still get all the benefits. That is why I teach yoga and DrumFit (a high energy aerobics class taught while drumming on yoga balls) and practice aerial and PoleFit (pole dance-style fitness class) and hooping. I am not one for long workouts in the gym or weight lifting, but the low-dose, high-effective body movements are a fun way to compete with yourself and, again, do not take up a lot of time, which I love. You start in a plank position and slowly lower into a push up for a five-count and slow lift for a five count back to plank. Then, just repeat until you can't do it anymore. Do the same for squats and pull-ups. Then try to beat your total the following day.

Don't underestimate the power of a to-do list. When my schedule is hectic and I know I have a million things to do, I make a list and for momentum, I add a couple quick and easy items to the list that I can bang out quick just to have the satisfaction of crossing it off the list. It is surprisingly therapeutic and gives you that sense of accomplishment, boosting your energy for the next task.

If and when you find yourself getting overwhelmed, pause, take a breath, and place your hand on your chest. There is an immense power in touch and that simple gesture can help to bring you back from the brink of panic.

In the event of a sudden panic attack, say out loud:

Five things that you can see,

Four things you can feel (touch them as you say what they are),

Three things you can hear,

Two things you can smell,

One thing you can taste.

Focusing your energy with intention helps to calm the mind and relax the breath so that you can regain your composure quickly and effectively.

Taking this further, I would like to introduce you to the power of tapping. Tapping is a simple technique that can be done anywhere on your own in a physical sense or visualized in a pinch. The beauty of tapping is that it is most effective in the moment, so as soon as a negative feeling or thought arises, you can start to release it and reprogram your thoughts with positive intentions by tapping on the meridian points (energy highways accessing different areas of the body).

Meridian Tapping Guide

When we think about optimal health, emotional barriers are too often over looked. Emotional health is just as important as physical health to promote ideal healing for the body. Tapping can play a very effective role in achieving emotional health and balance. Removing negative emotions can improve overall health, increase creativity, reduce food craving, eliminate pain, promote positive thinking, build confidence and help to achieve your goals. Tapping is a form of psychological acupressure. It is based on the same energy meridians that have been used in traditional acupuncture to treat physical and emotional ailments for over five thousand years, but without the use of needles. Begin by identifying a specific problem, concern or worry. This could be a traumatic event, addiction, insecurity or form of pain. Using the fingertips of one or both hands, tap energy onto specific meridians on the head and chest while you think about your specific problem and voice positive affirmations. Most meridian points exist on both sides of the body so you do not need to worry about what hand to use and can switch back and forth between sides if you choose to. While the number of taps is not critical, it is ideal to tap for the length of time that it takes to complete one full breath cycle – inhale and exhale.

Voicing positive affirmations while tapping the energy points allows the mind to clear the emotional block from your body's bioenergy system, restoring your mind and body's balance, which is essential for optimal health and the healing of both physical mental ailments. It is most beneficial to physically tap each point with your fingertips but what if something comes up while you are driving or in public? Simply run through the same technique silently to yourself while visualizing the tapping and then do the physical tapping and voice the affirmations out loud when you have a moment alone. It is always best to address our emotions immediately as they arise.

As we have discussed, your consistent thoughts mirror your reality. You succeed at what you give your attention to, including negative thought patterns. How you view the world around you is a reflection of your consistent thoughts. Tapping and affirmations helps to retrain your brain to more positive and productive thought patterns and beliefs.

TAPPING POINTS

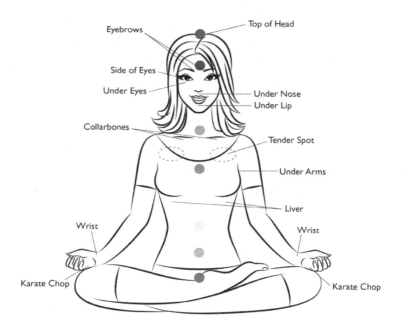

Eyebrows

Top of Head

Side of Eyes

Under Eyes

Under Nose

Under Lip

Collarbones

Tender Spot

Under Arms

Liver

Wrist

Wrist

Karate Chop

Karate Chop

Your affirmations will be personal and unique to the moment but allow me to offer you some samples that I use frequently for my clients and myself.

Starting with the karate chop, use the tips of your fingers on the opposite hand to tap the meridian point shown in the diagram above and recite a similar phrase filling in the blank with a suitable sentence for you.

Example

- Even though <u>I have allowed my fear to get in the way of my success</u>, I truly and completely love and accept myself.
- Even though <u>I have all this pain</u>, I truly and completely love and accept myself.
- Even though <u>I struggle with this memory</u>, I truly and completely love and accept myself.
- Then, starting at the top of your head and working your way down through each point, repeat your release statements.

Example

- I release myself from the belief that I do not have what it takes to be successful.

- I release myself from the belief that I am not enough.
- I release myself from the belief that I do not have the strength to overcome my pain.
- I release myself from the belief that I am limited by my past.
- Seal the session by tapping an open palm at heart center and offering yourself some loving and supportive "I" statements.

Example

- I am worthy of good in my life
- I am a beautiful, confident and determined person
- I am intelligent
- I have the power to overcome my past and truly heal

If this is starting to look familiar, it is because I have offered you these statements throughout the book. At the end of each chapter there are very intentionally placed affirmations. You may not believe it in this moment, but they are all true for you! Allow each of them to be your truth.

Embrace your power.

Guided Meditations

Follow the links below for access to three of my guided meditations. My meditation practice has changed multiple times over the years. When I was first teaching myself to meditate, I needed soothing music to keep me in the moment and really struggled to find a guided meditation that I enjoyed. As my practice developed, I found the music distracting and chose to use green noise instead. Green noise is similar to white noise (that fuzzy sound of an old T.V. or dead air on the radio), but it sounds more like nature – wind and crashing waves. More recently, I have preferred to meditate in silence and I come out of my meditative state by becoming aware of the natural sounds of my surrounding. Each of the guided scripts below are recorded using only my voice. This allows you the freedom to test what works best for you at your current stage of your practice and to alter it each time you listen. You can play relaxing music while you listen, you may choose to search a green noise track on YouTube or simple keep them as they are. Whatever you decide is perfect.

Healing Visualization

https://soundcloud.com/amlera/healing-visualization/s-BlzFg

Pain Management Relaxation

https://soundcloud.com/amlera/pain-management-relaxation/s-fXKFk

Self-Esteem Relaxation

https://soundcloud.com/amlera/self-esteem-meditation/s-q6aVb

Letting Go Full Moon Ritual

Start by writing down everything that you wish to let go of on small individual pieces of paper. It can be thought, feeling, person, event, anything that causes you pain and you wish to let go. Recite the intention statement below and release yourself from each item by burning the paper under the full moon. Safely discard of the ashes.

This full moon, I release that which no longer serves me. I release trauma and pain. I release the blocks that have kept me from connecting to the divine. I cut the cord connecting me to the trauma of my past lives. I start new today, free from guilt, hurt, and self-bondage that keeps me from manifesting the life that I desire.

In conjunction with these exercises, be sure to incorporate intention setting. This can be done at any point throughout the day as often as you need. You can set one intention for your overall day, one for an upcoming meeting or promotion, one for your practice or workout. The idea is to get into the habit of positive self-talk and goal setting. Invest in you. Be your biggest cheerleader because, as we have already discovered, our beliefs are being projected and mirrored back in our reality, so let's make it work with and for us in a way that honors our true self, brightens our path and leads us to the life we dreamed of.

How to stop time: Kiss.

How to travel in time: Read.

How to escape time: Music.

How to feel time: Write.

How to release time: Breathe.

Chapter 11:

Endless Beauty

*Y*ou have heard the saying, fix your thinking and your problems will fix themselves, but what does that even mean? We already know that telling ourselves we are fine when we are not is part of the problem, so how do we fix our thinking to fix our problems? First, we have to understand how we identify ourselves. Philosopher Charles Horton Cooley wrote, "I am not what you think I am, I am not what I think I am, I am what I think, you think I am." We have all these perceptions of who we think we should be and what we think we should want or achieve that we have no idea who we actually are or what we really want. We live our lives in autopilot, simply coasting through to the next phase and don't even realize what we are missing.

Take a look at where you are right now in your life and on your current path. Let's start with your career. Start with where you are currently and look at yourself in five to ten years, climbing the ladder in your current position. Is that where you want to be? Is that the life you really want for yourself, or are you content to settle for it as a "good enough" option? What about your current relationship status? What is your dream scenario in five years? In ten years? If you continue as you are, do you see yourself achieving those goals? If the answer is "no," then you need a new path. If you are unsure, the answer is probably no.

I encourage you to really sit with this. We allow ruts to form and barriers to build in our lives. We think that we are protecting ourselves from disappointment or rejection, but we are actually holding ourselves back. We reject and suppress ourselves before anyone else can. We follow suit, coasting through life and never really allow ourselves to shine. It is no wonder our hair is falling out. Our bodies and minds are not being fully nurtured and honored in order to facilitate growth.

Take a closer look at your life and ask yourself, "Is this what I really want, is it what I think I should want, or is it what others want for me?" I spent years thinking that one day I would get married and have children. I always saw myself having a big family, but as I got older, I realized that it wasn't that I wanted children, but rather that I always assumed I would have them because that is what is expected. The more I thought about it, the more I realized, maybe motherhood wasn't my path. Maybe this wasn't what I really wanted for my life. I started to ask myself why I wanted kids and the real answer was that I didn't. The older I got, the surer I was that I had made a decision based on societal expectations and what my family considered to be key elements of a happy, successful life.

As my older sisters got married and started having children of their own, I remember feeling relieved because it meant that my father had experienced walking his daughter down the aisle and my mother got the grandchildren that she always wanted. It took the pressure off of me needing to provide that for them. I wouldn't be letting anyone down if I decided not to get married or have children. No one ever told me I had to get married and have children in order to be happy, but that was an expectation I put on myself. Once I allowed myself the time and freedom to understand if being a mother was something I actually wanted or something I expected I would want, I discovered that I just assumed I should want it.

In reality, I am open to all the universe has to offer me, but at this time in my life, I know that children are not something that I want for myself. That choice alone comes with many stigmas. While I love children and would make an amazing mother, the fact that I can have children does not mean that I should. I am told regularly that I either don't know what I am talking about, that I haven't met the right person, or that I will change my mind. Maybe that's true, or maybe I have just given myself the time to get to know me and be able to live unapologetically as myself. Perhaps one day I will decide that I do want to have a child. One thing is for sure, I have allowed myself the time to identify my "why."

When I was younger, if you had asked me why I wanted kids, I could have given a list of responses; to have someone to care for me when I get old, I am really good with kids, everyone tells me that I would be a good mom, kids are cute, it's just what you do at a certain age. Once I relieved myself of the pressure of thinking that I had to have children by a certain age, I realized that I did not like my why. My responses seemed more like excuses to me than reasons.

With ever decision that I make, I ask myself why I want it. It is so simple yet so effective in getting to know yourself on a deeper level and provides such clarity in my decisions.

What do you think that would feel like for you? Are you living for what you really want or what you feel you should want? Can you identify your why?

Let's take this a little deeper. What are your thoughts telling you about yourself? How are you remembering past events? Remember, we have all experienced trauma and it affects us in many ways. Are you able to look back on one specific traumatic event that occurred for you? Go back as far as you need, but pick the event that first jumps out in your mind when you read the word trauma. You are probably able to remember specific details about the event – where you were, what you were wearing, exactly how it felt in each moment. Perhaps you are feeling that again now as you think about it. Jump forward to where you are today as you are, sitting and reading this book. Is there a part of that experience that you can look back on with genuine gratitude?

Our past experiences help shape our future. We are so much stronger for having gone through these things. Can you for a moment, separate the victim from the lesson? How are you better, stronger, more intelligent now than you were before that event? List all the ways in which you have rebuilt your life in order to move forward. Are you able to forgive them?

If that brought about anger or resentment for you, remember, forgiveness is for you. When you get to the point where you are able to forgive someone for their wrongdoing, you are releasing yourself from the hurt you have been carrying. Set yourself free. You do not have to rebuild a relationship with everyone you forgive. You don't even have to tell them you forgive them, but if you can find a way to forgive for yourself, you will find peace. Finding peace does not mean the situation is not still toxic, it just means it no longer has a hold on you.

The best way to find this forgiveness is to look for the lesson in the hurt: What did you gain from this? I am telling you that you are better for having experienced it; can you identify how? Praise yourself for your survival and strength. You are truly remarkable. Forgive so that you can free yourself from the hurt that has kept you stuck in a cycle of pain. Without even realizing it, we project our insecurities into our everyday lives. We attract what we think we deserve. We accept the love that we think we deserve. If you do not see your strength, beauty, value, and worth, how can you expect anyone else to?

I was in a group meditation the first time my need for validation was pointed out to me. We were talking about trusting our gut, listening to our inner navigator – our instinct – hearing the voice of our spirit guides. I mentioned that I second-guessed myself and that I was told that if I could overcome the fear, then I could be very powerful. I told a story about how often I am told that my instincts are strong and powerful. She stopped me and asked, "Why do you need someone else to validate that for you?" She pointed out that instead of me telling her how I felt or what I believed my strengths to be, I was only referring to what others thought of me. I had not even realized that in the way I was telling my story, I was giving up my power to others. Instead of standing firm in what I know and feel to be true about myself, I discussed what others had said about me. As if that somehow made it more valid, more real. Why did I need someone else to validate my strengths? Why were others' opinions of myself more credible than my own? I had let my fear and insecurities surface without even realizing. I was projecting them in what I perceived in the moment as an empowering statement, but how empowering is it if someone else has to validate it for you? Every one of us has a strong intuition, a gut instinct, and untapped wisdom. Some of us are just more open and willing to listen to it.

There are plenty of theories to support that each of us has a sixth sense, but many people believe that it is a gift that only a few individuals possess. The reality is that we all have the ability to tap into our sixth sense, but we have suppressed it or allowed it to lay dormant for so long that we have forgotten how. Few have allowed it to be active while the rest of us have shut it off out of fear, self-doubt or lack of necessity. Many believe that the sixth sense is only about seeing dead people or accessing the other side, but it is so much more than that. Our sixth sense is a trusted instinct, a gut feeling. It is linked to survival.

Back when our species had to hunt for our food, we had to rely heavily on our instincts to tell us if danger was near. We could predict weather patterns and gauge pregnancy cycles on the moon. As we evolved, our need for the survival instinct has minimized. We have comfortable homes for shelter. We no longer have to hunt for our food or worry about when, where, and if our next meal is coming. We rely on apps for the weather. We have technology that essentially caters to our every need, right down to our sense of security with surveillance systems easily accessible.

Our need for our sixth sense has diminished, and our minds have evolved with the times, allowing it to sit quietly untapped in the back of our minds. Society continues to teach us that we need to search for answers from outside sources causing us to second guess ourselves, questioning if we really know what is best. We rely on our other five senses to experience our physical world because that is all we think we need to know. This is why "animal instinct" is so much more common and accepted. Animals haven't evolved in the same way and still rely on their survival instincts or sixth sense. If everything is made up of energy then we are all connected and have great untapped knowledge inside of us. Are you ready to tap into those answers? Are you open to your own abilities? Can you allow yourself to trust your navigator?

The degree to which a person can grow is directly proportional to the amount of truth they can accept about themselves without running away.

I am the creator of my reality. I am complete. I am change.

Chapter 12:

"Beliefs"

There will always be obstacles standing in the way of what we tell ourselves we really want. This is the universe's way of gauging your growth. How much do you really want it? How hard are you willing to work to achieve your dreams? Do you actually want your "dreams" or are you telling yourself that you should? Do you assume you will be happier if you achieved it yet subconsciously sabotage yourself because it is easier to stay stuck? Do you continue passing blame and making excuses for why things cannot be easy? Life happens. Work gets in the way. The children are sick. There has been a family emergency. A sudden passing of a loved one. An unexpected illness. A soccer practice. Ballet recital. Car trouble. Health issues. The list is endless. There will always be a million reasons not to achieve your dreams – countless reasons why there just are not enough hours in the day to devote to something as superficial as growing your hair back.

Let's get real, it's more than that and you know it. You want more for yourself and you deserve more for yourself, so why can't you get out of your own way? What would it mean to you to actually achieve what it is that you say you want? Why do you think it is easier to just stay where you are? Sure, there is security and comfort in the mundane and familiar. There is reliability in that which you already know but if the meaning of life is to experience all that we can while we are here then we owe it to ourselves to break the barriers that we have built for ourselves. You can keep telling yourself that if you just had more time, or a better paying job, or a more supportive partner, or if your car/school/home was just paid off, then you would be able to commit more time to you, but the truth is, none of that matters. The only thing that has to change in order for you to be where you want to be is for you to stop the cycle of lies that you have been telling yourself. Even if all of those things miraculously resolved themselves tomorrow, there would be a whole new list of reasons why now just isn't the right time.

Each day is comprised of 86,400 seconds. Think about that in terms of dollars. What if each morning $86,400 were deposited into your bank account and whatever you didn't use at the end of the day was lost? You cannot carry it over into the next day; it does not get saved anywhere and can never be recovered. How would you use that money? The universe replenishes our account every day in the form of time and we choose how and if we will use it.

Notice I specifically said choose. Everything in your life is a choice – yes, there are things that occur that are out of our control, but it is completely up to us how we handle those situations and what we do with those new experiences and information moving forward. It is so easy – and dare I say, lazy – to just look at all the negative that surrounds our lives and let it take over. It's easy to say, "I had a bad day, so I am going to shut out the world and stay in bed for the next three days." Don't get me wrong, we all need to acknowledge when we need time to recharge, and if that means doing nothing, by all means, take advantage of that, but make sure it serves a purpose. Remember when we discussed validating your feelings but not living in them? Take your time, but make a mental note of what that experience means to you, why it had the effect that it did, what you need in order to move forward in peace and what you can take from it in order to better your life tomorrow.

Our "beliefs" are what forms our reality. I use the quotes because I am not referring to our religious beliefs. I am talking about our personal beliefs. Our thoughts about ourselves that manifest into deep-rooted beliefs that we may not even realize that we are sending out to the universe and in turn are being mirrored back in reality as we know it. Positive self-talk is a wonderful start, but how much of what you say to yourself or others do you actually believe and feel supported by? Are you speaking your truth or speaking in a way you "think" you should? There is a big difference here. Will you allow yourself the strength and courage that it takes to turn your beliefs on their head. The more we treat ourselves with uncertainty and judgment, the more susceptible we become to those obstacles being cycled through our reality.

For example, if you are constantly telling yourself, "I really want this upcoming promotion. I am totally ready for it and would be great in the role, but there are so many more qualified applicants, I probably won't get it," chances are that you won't get it. You may think that you are just being modest or realistic, but you have unconsciously set up a barrier. You have told the universe when to step in and what to give you, and it delivered.

We spend our whole lives developing certain beliefs about ourselves without even realizing that we are doing it. We set ourselves up for failure and then question why we failed. It's a vicious cycle because we see it as confirmation that our insecurities are true, when really we are being treated the way we have asked. Can you identify the lesson in the self- deprecation? How is it really serving you?

The underlining factor in all of our obstacles is fear. Fear of failure, embarrassment, reinforced insecurities and disappointment but also fear of success. This fear we carry so deeply is manifesting in our hair loss. You may think that's ridiculous. Why would anyone be afraid to succeed but there are many reasons. With success comes responsibility and accountability that you may not feel you are truly equipped for because it means a lot of hard work and long hours, which you may think, "I'm doing that already, why would that scare me?" Maybe it takes you out of your comfort zone, sure you can handle it, but you aren't sure if you want to or better yet, if it will all be worth it. What if you put in all that work and effort and fail and don't have anything to fall back on? It is easier to just stay where you are right? It's safe and reliable, so no point in messing with a good thing. It's too risky. Perhaps what you are really thinking is, "Who am I to deserve this?" "What qualities or experience do I have to make me worthy of success?" "No one would take me seriously, I'm not credible enough." What you are really saying is that you are not enough and that thought in itself is scary, but I am here to assure you that you are more than enough, and you can overcome your fears and misconceptions because that is all they are. It is not who you are.

As we discussed earlier, we all have trauma. We all have fears and doubts but we also all have experiences and knowledge that makes us unique and qualified for greatness. You can overcome. Our soul has chosen the life that we need in order to experience, adapt, learn, and grow. A beautiful song lyric by First Aid Kit is, "I'd rather be broken than empty." Broken is feeling, broken is mendable, broken has the potential to keep going. Although we may perceive ourselves to be empty, empty is when we stop feeling, stop learning, stop growing, stop living. We are all a little broken in our own way but that again is what makes us so special and what gives us the ability to help others. We all have different experience and expertise, and we all have knowledge that we can gain from one another.

Be mindful of the words and phrases you chose to describe yourself. Be deliberate in your desires and expectations.

What is it that you are really asking the universe for? Are you open to receiving it? Are you open to all that it has to offer to you for your growth and betterment? Can you be honest with yourself about what you really want and confident enough to say it without telling yourself that it's cocky or self-assured? Being modest isn't serving you. You don't have to dim your light from shining in others eyes, hand them sunglasses. If people are intimidated by your strength or success, it is a weakness in them, not you.

Find your dream and then live every moment in pursuit of it. Let every decision you make from now on to be in honor of that dream.

Greatness is small things done well; take one step at a time. Do one small thing each day and do it well!

"When you want to succeed as bad as you want to breathe, then you'll be successful."
– Eric Thomas

I am a warrior. I am intelligent. I have purpose. I will achieve my dreams.

Chapter 13:

Conclusion

*B*e passionate about your craft and create work that will live beyond your journey here on earth. Say goodbye to the bad things. Say goodbye to all the times you felt lost or alone. Say goodbye to all the scrapes, bruises and heartache, all the times it was a "no" instead of a "yes." Remember, they didn't leave you; it wasn't a missed opportunity. You are enough. As we heal and grow, our energy grows. It is asking others to rise up but not everyone is willing to go where they would grow. You may not be willing to see it but the universe has moved it out of your way to make room for something better. Give gratitude for the experiences that brought you the strength and knowledge to get you to where you are today. Hold on to the good, which makes you smile and brings love and light into your heart and adds a bounce in your step. Move forward each day with pride, love, acceptance, and appreciation for all the good you have made room for in your life with your healing. You are never "too old" and it is never "too late." Each day that you wake up is a new opportunity for a fresh start, a new deposit of 86,400 seconds. Use them to build a life you don't need a vacation from. Wake each day in pursuit of your bliss. Honor your true self in the way you deserve. Believe in yourself so much that it has no choice but to materialize.

You are destined for greatness and have all my love and support in the process.

If you are feeling depressed, you are living in the past, if you feel anxious, you are living in the future. It is when you are living in the present that you feel at peace.

"Figure out who you are and do it on purpose"
– Dolly Parton

Should you have any questions or would just like to touch base, please feel free to leave me a message at amlera@live.com.

I love to hear from you and would be honored to continue to work with you further.

You are abundant. You are worthy. You are certain. You are free. You are light.

Blessings to a beautiful soul. xo

Yours truly,

Amanda Lera

Acknowledgments

To my lovely Lisa Borkovich: How do I even begin to thank you? I truly believe that I spent much of my early years ignoring my spirit guides, so they sent me you in their place. I cannot even put into words the amount of love, respect, and gratitude I have for you. I came to you years ago as an absolute last resort. I was a skeptic, but had tried everything and to no avail, but you so lovingly, so genuinely, and open-mindedly accepted me into your home and gave me the most amazing gift. Your gentle guidance and wisdom gave me the key to unlocking my true potential and power. I will never forget the hours we spent in your front room or all the knowledge you graced me with during your teaching. You don't even know this, but you continue to be my North Star. You see, over the years whenever I am going through a rough time personally or am on the precipice of transformation, and question whether or not I am on the right path, I run into you. We live in the same neighborhood, yet our paths cross so infrequently. Then, just as I need you, even when I don't know that I do, there you are. Your simple presence – whether it be a conversation in the grocery store, a quick hello at a festival, a smile and nod as we spot each other across the street or the handful of times that I've been driving and pass you walking, however big or small our interaction – you are my guide, my sign from the universe reassuring me that I've made it to the other side of whatever I was going through and that I am where I need to be. You were the first step on my path to healing and I am truly blessed to have met you. I can only hope that the reader of this book experiences the same sense of security, calm, unconditional love, and self-empowerment that I get from you.

Kasia and Dan, the word powerful comes to mind a million times over when I think of you both. You have been the answer to so many of the questions that I have asked the universe. Much like Lisa, you both came to me at a time when I needed ... something. I wasn't even sure what it was until I met you. I will never forget our first meeting when Dan apologized for leading me too far. He nodded and said I wasn't ready, and he made that okay for me. Our next meeting was even more powerful, and I cannot thank you enough, for not only leading me down that path, but for so lovingly holding my hand the whole way. I am so grateful for the work we have done together and look forward to many more magical journeys with you both. Much love.

Thank you to Angela Lauria and The Author Incubator's team, as well as to David Hancock and the Morgan James Publishing team for helping me bring this book to print.

Thank You

This may be the end of the book, but it is only the beginning of our journey together. Beginnings always hide themselves in endings. ;)

As an expression of my deepest respect and gratitude I would like to offer you the following gifts.

Email me at amlera@live.com with the subject line "I want more," and you will receive:

- A beautiful colored chart for How to Unblock Your Chakras
- Access to my three-part yoga and mindfulness series with some quick and gentle flows for individuals of all levels, followed by a soothing guided meditation and breathing exercise

- My introduction to tapping, which will help you take your practice deeper

And don't forget to include your name and availability to schedule your free thirty-minute one-to-one consultation.

About the Author

$\mathcal{A}$manda Lera is a social ser- vice worker and founder of Just Breathe, a fitness and holistic health practice. She studies and teaches a wide variety of fitness modalities, including yoga, acro, suspension yoga, DrumFit, and Zumba, and has a strong interest in biomechanics, low-dose, high-effective 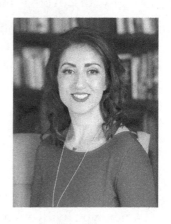 training. She offers natural, gentle treatments to her clients for a growing list of health benefits and healing properties, resulting in the resolve of a range of ailments. Amanda has led a number of mindfulness talks and workshops across Ontario.

In 2014, when Amanda first started to notice random patches of hair falling out, she set out on a mission to solve what, to her, was the worst thing to happen. Shallow? Maybe, but her hair was her security blanket. After countless doctor visits, expensive treatments, medications, diets, and exercises with no diagnosis or resolve, Amanda not only discovered the cause of her hair loss, but developed a solution to grow it back and prevent it from happening again. After two years of struggles, each patch falling out being bigger than the last, Amanda now has complete regrowth in all areas and has gone years without a recurring episode.

Amanda devotes her time to helping others like her achieve the same lasting results. When not working, Amanda can be found collecting certifications for her latest interests and spending time outdoors. During the summer, you will often find Amanda at the Bay Front reading, doing yoga, and going for walks with her tortoise, Darius Redfoot.

CPSIA information can be obtained
at www.ICGtesting.com
Printed in the USA
JSHW030154190620
6258JS00003B/208